YOUR KNOWLEDGE HAS VALUE

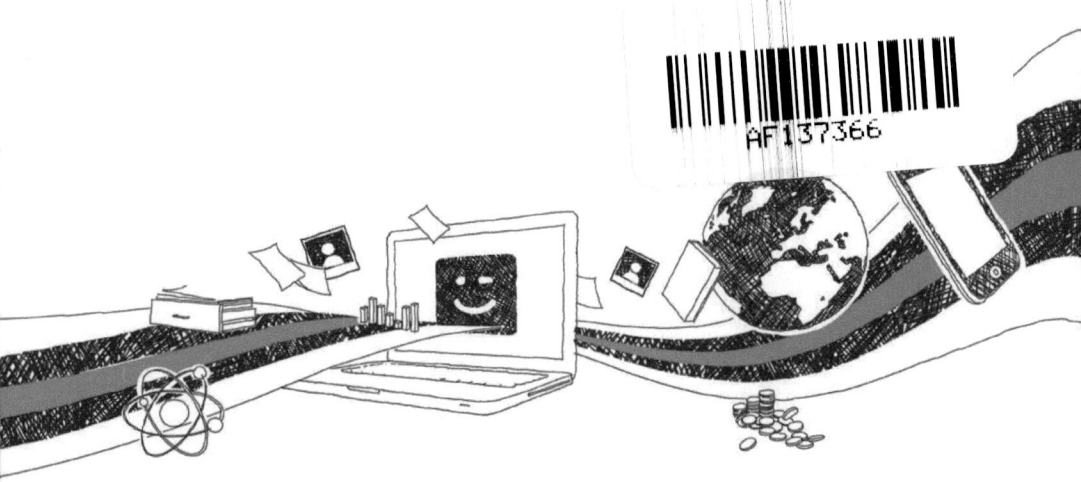

- We will publish your bachelor's and
  master's thesis, essays and papers

- Your own eBook and book -
  sold worldwide in all relevant shops

- Earn money with each sale

Upload your text at www.GRIN.com
and publish for free

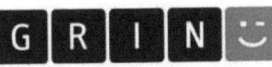

The Influence of Pharmaceutical Ads. Strategies, Psychology, and Ethics in Medicine Marketing

KEIFARI ASGHAR

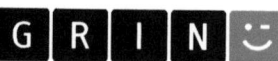

Bibliographic information published by the German National Library:

The German National Library lists this publication in the National Bibliography; detailed bibliographic data are available on the Internet at http://dnb.dnb.de.

ISBN: 9783346978721
This book is also available as an ebook.

© GRIN Publishing GmbH
Trappentreustraße 1
80339 München

All rights reserved

Print and binding: Books on Demand GmbH, Norderstedt, Germany
Printed on acid-free paper from responsible sources.

The present work has been carefully prepared. Nevertheless, authors and publishers do not incur liability for the correctness of information, notes, links and advice as well as any printing errors.

GRIN web shop: https://www.grin.com/document/1400559

University of Szeged

Faculty of Pharmacy

Pharmacy operation, management

Pharmaceuticals Advertising, Advertising Psychology

Thesis

Made by:

Dr. Keifari Asghar

Szeged

2023

Table of Contents

1. Abstract

Pharmaceutical ads play a big role where medicine marketing and psychology meet in today's fast-moving world of spreading information. This study dives deep into this connection, looking at the strategies and psychology behind medication ads. It uses real research, examples, and careful thinking to show how these ads can change how people think and act when it comes to medicines.

It's not just about saying good things about medicines. The study also looks at how these ads can affect our choices, sometimes in tricky ways. It also talks about when it's not okay to use sneaky tricks to get people to pick certain health products. Nowadays, we have lots of information, so these ads mixed with psychology can really affect how people decide about their health. This study wants to make this whole process clearer and more honest so that people can make good choices about their health.

On another note, things like radio, TV, and the internet have made it very easy to share information about medicines. But this has also raised questions about whether it's okay to directly advertise medical products to the public. There are rules in the European Union (EU) about how medicines can be advertised. Hungary follows these rules and has its own as well. They even have a special centre to help with all this, and they want to make sure medicines are reliable, people are safe, and everything is fair.

Upon the culmination of the research, a questionnaire was administered to both pharmacists and patients. What we found from their answers is that everyone agrees - they think advertising for non-prescription medications is good. They also think it's important to have strong rules and control over these ads.

2. Introduction

In our fast-changing world, where information spreads through advanced channels, pharmaceutical advertising is at a crucial point. It's where strategies to market medicines meet the complex world of advertising psychology. This mix is fascinating and powerful. It can shape what people think, how they feel, and what they do. This doesn't just affect the pharmaceutical companies; it's also important for the people who use and prescribe medicines.

Pharmaceutical advertising has changed a lot because of new technology and how people behave. pharmaceutical companies want to reach their audience and share important medical information. Advertising psychology helps them understand how to persuade people, trigger emotions, and influence choices. This isn't just about selling things; it's also about ethics and what's right when persuading people.

The study aims to understand how pharmaceutical advertising and advertising psychology work together. It looks at the strategies used in pharmaceutical ads and figures out why they work on people's minds. This is done by studying real examples, doing research, and carefully looking at advertising methods. The goal is to give a complete picture of how advertising psychology affects what people think and do when it comes to medicine.

Advertising psychology isn't just about selling products. It's about understanding how people make choices, what biases they might have, and what emotions can influence them. When exploring how this works in the context of medicine, we'll also talk about the ethics of using persuasive techniques to influence healthcare decisions. The study aims to add to the conversation about how we communicate medical information, make informed choices, and empower patients.

In today's world, where information spreads easily online, the mix of pharmaceutical advertising and advertising psychology can have a big impact on public health. It can shape the decisions people make about their health. By studying this relationship closely, we hope to uncover what drives pharmaceutical advertising and how we can create a more informed and ethical way of making healthcare choices. [1]

3. History of Pharmaceutical Advertising

The history of pharmaceutical advertising is like a story with many layers, filled with new ideas, changes in society, and the evolving understanding of healthcare. This section delves into key historical milestones that have shaped the advertising of pharmaceuticals, providing insights into the gradual fusion of medical communication and advertising techniques.

3.1. Ancient Beginnings: Sharing Remedies and Medical Wisdom

Throughout history, communities relied on oral traditions, symbols, and basic ways of sharing information about healing practices and remedies. Ancient civilizations like Egypt, Greece, and China used simple medical writings, inscriptions, and symbols to talk about the benefits of certain herbs, treatments, and practices. These early ways of spreading information laid the foundation for how medical knowledge and communication came together.

When calendars and writing came into use, it marked the start of recorded history. Knowledge was written on clay tablets with special signs and seals, which ancient Mesopotamian doctors used. In the Louvre Museum, there's a stone pillar with Hammurabi's Code, a set of laws from an ancient Babylonian king in the 18th century BCE. It had strict punishments, even cutting off body parts for deadly medical mistakes. [2]

3.2. Print Revolution and the Emergence of Medical Advertisements

The invention of the printing press in the 15th century was a big turning point in advertising history. It allowed for the mass production of books and pictures. This meant that medical books and ads for treatments could reach more people, giving them information about different ways to get better. The printing press also made it cheaper to print things on paper.

By the 17th century, newspapers and large printed sheets started showing ads for things like elixirs, tonics, and treatments that promised to cure many different illnesses. However, these early medical ads were often based on stories and didn't have strong scientific proof behind them. [3]

3.3. Industrialization and the Birth of Modern Pharmaceutical Advertising

The 19th century witnessed the industrial revolution and significant advancements in medicine, including the development of synthesized medications and the rise of pharmaceutical companies. With the increased production and availability of medicines, pharmaceutical manufacturers sought effective ways to reach wider audiences. The emergence of popular magazines and trade publications provided platforms for pharmaceutical advertisements to gain prominence. [4]

3.4. 20th Century and the Rise of Direct-to-Consumer Advertising

In recent decades, there has been a significant change in how consumers are involved in healthcare, which has led to many discussions about policies. This shift is similar to the early 1900s when people took care of their health, and most Pharmaceutical ads were aimed at consumers. The 20th century brought big changes to how pharmaceuticals were marketed because of new technology and rules. Radio, television, and later the internet made it possible to share medical information worldwide. In the mid-1900s, the United States saw the start of direct-to-consumer (DTC) advertising, where Pharmaceutical companies could talk directly to patients. This change led to debates about the ethics of promoting medical products to the public because healthcare decisions are complex. [5] [6]

3.5. Ethical and Regulatory Challenges

As pharmaceutical advertising developed, so did the concerns about ethics and rules related to it. There were worries about making exaggerated claims, not giving complete information, and influencing healthcare choices too much. To address these concerns, regulatory bodies like the Food and Drug Administration (FDA) in the United States and similar agencies in other countries started making rules to make sure pharmaceutical ads were accurate and fair.

The history of pharmaceutical advertising shows how it has changed over time because of new ways to communicate, what society expects, and the responsibility of Pharmaceutical companies. Looking at this history helps us understand the challenges and opportunities we face in the future when advertising medications while also following the rules of advertising psychology and ethical healthcare communication.

4. Pharmaceutical Advertising Regulations

4. 1. European Union Pharmaceutical Advertising Regulations

The European Union Pharmaceutical Advertising Regulations encompass a comprehensive set of rules and standards designed to regulate the advertising and promotion of pharmaceutical products within the EU member states. These regulations are vital to ensure the safety, transparency, and ethical conduct of pharmaceutical advertising campaigns, while also promoting fair competition within the industry.

4.1.1. EU Directive 2001/83/EC and Regulation (EC) No 726/2004

Directive 2001/83/EC serves as the cornerstone of regulatory frameworks governing the authorization and marketing of pharmaceutical products within the European Union (EU). This directive lays down fundamental principles for the advertising and promotion of medicinal products across member states. It highlights the imperative need for effective and comprehensive monitoring in the advertising of pharmaceuticals, as elucidated in Article 97, emphasizing rigorous oversight. Additionally, Article 98 mandates that Marketing Authorization Holders (MAHs) establish a scientific service responsible for disseminating information about medicinal products and ensuring strict compliance with decisions made by monitoring authorities. Importantly, the directive refrains from providing specific guidelines for the control of pharmaceutical advertising, granting Member States (MS) a degree of autonomy in tailoring their monitoring procedures.

The incorporation of the European Directive into national legal frameworks has led to a diverse array of domestic adaptations and regulatory guidelines throughout Member States, resulting in varying approaches to the monitoring and control of pharmaceutical promotion. Depending on the MS, oversight of pharmaceutical advertising compliance may be conducted by government agencies, national competent authorities, or through self-regulatory mechanisms. The concept of "self-regulation" allows for the delegation of monitoring and control activities, especially in cases where no national competent authority has been designated. Often, this delegation extends to entities such as national pharmaceutical industry associations, multi-stakeholder groups, or the pharmaceutical companies themselves, which establish their unique codes of conduct and hold the authority to assess and approve pharmaceutical advertisements. [7]

4.1.2. EU Directive 2005/29/EC

At the European Union level, the UCP Directive, officially known as Directive 2005/29/EC, regulates commercial practices directed at consumers across various sectors, encompassing products and services such as medicines, medical devices, and food. Specifically, the UCP Directive establishes a comprehensive prohibition against deceptive and forceful advertising. Under this directive, advertising is considered deceptive if it contains false information or utilizes presentation techniques that could potentially mislead the average consumer, regardless of the accuracy of the information, leading them to make a transactional decision they otherwise would not have made. Aggressive commercial practices, as outlined in the directive, encompass advertising tactics that exert undue influence or pressure on consumers, significantly impeding their ability to make well-informed decisions. [8]

4.1.3. Directive 2006/114/EC3

Directive 2006/114/EC aims to protect businesses from misleading advertising by other businesses, similar to unfair commercial practices. It sets the rules for when comparative advertising is allowed. It's important to note that these rules on comparative advertising, as described in Directive 2006/114/EC, go beyond advertising to consumers. This directive defines "misleading advertising" as any type of advertising that can potentially trick the people it's meant for, whether they are the intended audience or others. Deceptive advertising, because it's misleading, can impact how people make economic choices and can also harm competitors or have the potential to harm them.

When these European Union legal rules become part of a country's laws, how they are enforced can be different from one country to another. Various methods are used for making sure these rules are followed. In some Member States, businesses can start legal actions against their competitors directly if they think these rules are being violated. But in other countries, only regulatory authorities are allowed to initiate legal actions in such cases.

It's also important to understand that each country might have its own additional rules that apply to both general consumer advertising practices and advertising campaigns for specific products or services. These extra restrictions add to the overall set of rules that govern advertising in the European Union. [9]

4.1.5. Advertising to the General Public

Currently, Article 88 of Directive 2001/83/EC, which lays out the regulations for pharmaceutical advertising, forbids the direct advertising of prescription-only medicines to consumers and Direct-to-consumer (DTC) advertising of prescription medicines is generally prohibited in the EU. There are exceptions for over-the-counter (OTC) medicines, but even these must comply with strict regulations. [10]

4.2. Governmental Institutes Regulating Pharmaceuticals and Pharmacies in Hungary

Hungarian Act on Medicinal Products: Hungary follows the EU framework for pharmaceutical advertising but also has its own national regulations, outlined in the Hungarian Act on Medicinal Products. This act is aligned with EU directives and provides specific guidelines for pharmaceutical advertising.

4.2.1. Approval by Nemzeti Népegészségügyi és Gyógyszerészeti Központ" (NNGYK), "National Center for Public Health and Pharmacy

On July 20, 2023, the Hungarian government issued Decree No. 333/2023, establishing the "Nemzeti Népegészségügyi és Gyógyszerészeti Központ" (NNGYK), which translates to the "National Center for Public Health and Pharmacy" in English. Concurrently, the "Országos Gyógyszerészeti és Élelmezés-egészségügyi Intézet" (OGYÉI), known as the "National Institute of Pharmacy and Food Health" in English, merged into the "Nemzeti Népegészségügyi Központ" (NNK), or "National Public Health Centre" in English, on August 1, 2023.

As of August 1, 2023, all functions previously carried out by OGYÉI have been transferred to NNGYK, which now assumes full responsibility for these essential roles and activities.

Due to the fact that the medication is a unique product, it is placed in a separate category that requires a more detailed review and control of all relevant information. This includes brochures for pharmaceutical products designed for healthcare professionals and advertising aimed at non-professionals. In accordance with the specialized rules governing the advertising of medicinal products, formerly OGYÉI and from August 1, 2023, NNGYK is dedicated to maintaining the accuracy, consistency and validity of published information about these medications. [11] [12] [13]

1. The OGYÉI (March 1, 2015 - August 1, 2023)

The National Institute of Pharmacy and Nutrition (OGYÉI) was originally established and appointed by Government Decree 28/2005 on March 1, 2015.

OGYÉI functioned as a licensing authority for pharmaceutical and government administrative affairs, with its primary objective being the provision of safe, effective, and high-quality medicines to the general public in compliance with regulations. Additionally, OGYÉI held national responsibilities for the control of narcotics and served as Hungary's methodical and research institute in this field.

OGYÉI played a vital role in reviewing notifications related to the quality of pharmaceutical products and adverse medication reactions. It was also responsible for authorizing pharmaceutical products and ensuring the removal of defective batches that posed a threat to human health from the market. OGYÉI had the authority to grant manufacturing and distribution licenses for pharmaceutical products, as well as oversee parallel import activities while maintaining strict adherence to good manufacturing practices. The institute was actively involved in clinical, laboratory, and pharmacovigilance activities related to the development and marketing of medicinal products.

Furthermore, OGYÉI was tasked with authorizing and supervising clinical trials for investigational medicinal products, managing off-label indications, addressing individual demands for medicinal products, and overseeing the distribution of medicinal products. The institute also dedicated efforts to combat counterfeit and illegal pharmaceutical product distribution and actively participated in international collaborations to counteract counterfeit pharmaceuticals. OGYÉI contributed to the operation of the OMCL (Official Medicines Control Laboratory) network, a network of national laboratories that examine medicinal products under the supervision of the European Directorate for the Quality of Medicines and Healthcare (EDQM), focusing on the investigation of questionable medicinal products.

OGYÉI took on administrative responsibilities related to medication procurement and ensured that senior pharmacist officers supervised and coordinated the operations of pharmacies to guarantee the accurate supply of appropriate products. The institute was also responsible for preparing national and international publications, posters, and presentations. OGYÉI conducted quality assessments of pharmaceutical products, conducted necessary tests to provide expert opinions, and monitored pharmaceutical advertising compliance. [14] [15]

2. The NNK (2018 - August 1, 2023)

The National Center for Public Health (NNK) is a government institution in Hungary that receives funding from the central budget. It is distinguished by its structured economic organization and operates as a central administrative office. Established in 2018, NNK was designed to take on the role of the legal successor to the National Public Health and Medical Officer Service (ÁNTSZ). From December 2018 to August 1, 2023, the Chief National Medical Officer, Cecília Müller, served as the authorized leader of NNK. Additionally, she currently holds the position of the head of NNGYK.

NNK expanded its authority by assuming the responsibilities of the National Institute of Public Health and acquiring resources from the Ministry of State (EMMI). The centre had national authority in various areas, including public health, epidemiological safety, patient safety, health promotion, hospital hygiene, and licensing. It also oversaw the operations of medical and occupational health institutions.

The Chief National Medical Officer's role included professionally supervising entities designated to carry out public health and epidemiological functions for the Hungarian Defence Forces and law enforcement agencies.

The establishment of NNK significantly improved the rapid response capabilities for national epidemiological activities. [16] [17]

4.3. Pharmaceutical Advertising Laws in Hungary

Considering the unique role that medicinal products and medical aids play in maintaining health, disease prevention, treatment, and enhancing quality of life,

Recognizing that even successful disease prevention efforts may not eliminate individual disparities caused by illness and poor health, and that state regulations are necessary to ensure fairness, justice, and effectiveness in reducing these disparities,

Acknowledging the importance of efficiently allocating funds from the social security system and individual spending on medicinal products and medical aids as a societal priority,

Understanding that modernizing the field of Pharmacology is essential for a modern healthcare system, relying on both national traditions and international standards and practices,

Noting that the industrialization of medicinal product production, changing consumer habits and preferences, and advances in information technology have significantly altered the retail distribution of medicinal products,

Recognizing the state's responsibility to establish regulations that ensure a safe and timely supply of medicinal products to patients in appropriate locations,

Acknowledging that individuals who purchase medicinal products are often vulnerable due to illness and lack expertise in this area, and that stricter regulations are essential to protect consumers,

Keeping in mind that regulated competition in the retail supply of medicinal products benefits consumers by improving their access to medicinal products and the quality of care,

4.3.1. Act XCVIII of 2006

Act XCVIII of 2006 in Hungary is officially titled the "Medicines Thrift Act." This legislation plays a crucial role in governing the reliable and economically feasible supply of medicinal products and medical aids, along with the distribution of medicinal products. It also extends its applicability to medical devices that qualify as medical aids.

The Medicines Thrift Act covers important areas of regulating medicinal products, such as authorization, distribution, quality control, and safety. It follows the directives and standards set by the European Union for medicinal products. This act plays a crucial role in Hungary's healthcare and pharmaceutical regulations, making sure these vital healthcare elements work correctly and are properly supervised. [18] [19]

4.3.2. Decree no. 3/2009 (II. 25.)

The "3/2009 (II. 25.) EüM Decree" establishes comprehensive regulations governing the description of medicinal products and medical aids intended for human use. It also outlines the requirements for registering individuals engaged in information activities and regulates commercial practices targeting consumers in relation to medicinal products and medical aids.

Similarly, "Decree no. 3/2009 (II. 25.) of the Minister of Health," known as the "Promotional Decree," provides detailed guidelines regarding the promotion of medicinal products for human use and medical aids. This decree also covers the registration of individuals involved in promotional activities and governs commercial practices directed at consumers concerning medicinal products and medical aids. Notably, these provisions extend to medical devices that meet the criteria for classification as medical aids. [20]

4.3.3. Act XLVIII of 2008

Act XLVIII of 2008, also known as the "Advertisement Act," lays out important requirements and specific limits for commercial advertising activities. Its goal is to establish essential standards and boundaries to ensure responsible and ethical advertising practices. This act, which includes provisions related to competition law, aims to protect public health, especially that of young people, reduce disruptions to social order, and maintain fair market competition that benefits the economy and society. It regulates various aspects of business advertising, sponsorship, and associated codes of conduct.

This Act applies to people involved in business advertising activities, such as advertisers, advertising service providers, or publishers of advertisements, as well as to sponsorship and the codes of conduct related to these activities. Additional rules may be created for specific goods or communication methods related to business advertising activities through other laws or regulations.

In this Act, "business advertising" means any form of communication, information, or representation designed to promote the sale or use of movable property, services, immovable property, and intangible assets (excluding immovable property). It also covers efforts to make a business's name, designation, activities, or product names more popular. [21] [22]

4.3.4. The "XLVII of 2008 Law

The Act XLVIII of 2008, also known as the "Advertisement Act," is a comprehensive piece of legislation that outlines important rules and restrictions for commercial advertising activities. Its primary purpose is to establish essential standards and boundaries for commercial advertising to ensure responsible and ethical practices in advertising endeavors. This act also encompasses provisions related to competition law, with the overarching goal of protecting public health, especially that of young people, reducing disruptions to social order, and maintaining fair market competition that benefits the economy and society. It regulates various aspects of business advertising activities, sponsorship, and associated codes of conduct.

This Act applies to individuals involved in business advertising activities, including advertisers, advertising service providers, and publishers of advertisements, as well as to sponsorship and the codes of conduct associated with these activities. Special rules may be established for specific goods or communication methods related to business advertising activities through other statutes or implementing laws.

For the purposes of this Act, "business advertising" refers to any form of communication, information, or representation aimed at promoting the sale or use of tradeable movable property, services, immovable property, and intangible assets, excluding immovable property. It also includes efforts to popularize the name, designation, or activities of businesses or to enhance the recognition of goods or designations of goods.

The Act sets out requirements and limitations for advertising, sponsorship, and other commercial activities. Violations of these provisions may result in legal consequences.

This Act plays a significant role in shaping the landscape of commercial advertising and ensuring that it operates in an ethical and responsible manner, benefiting both businesses and consumers.

4.3.4. Act CLV of 1997

Act CLV of 1997 on Consumer Protection (**"Consumer Protection Act"**);

It's important to note that pharmaceutical companies operating in Hungary and the wider EU must navigate a complex regulatory landscape when it comes to advertising their products. This includes ensuring that their promotional materials comply with both EU-wide and national regulations.[23]

5. Advertising models

Advertising models are conceptual frameworks that help marketers and advertisers understand how communication and persuasion work in the context of promoting products or services.

These models provide insights into consumer behavior and guide the creation of effective advertising campaigns. Let's delve into some popular advertising models:

5.1 AIDA model

The AIDA model which stands for Attention, Interest, Desire, and Action, is a well-known marketing and advertising framework used in various industries, including pharmaceuticals. In the context of pharmaceutical advertising, the AIDA model can be applied as follows:

5.1.1. Attention (A)

This This phase focuses on the crucial task of grabbing the audience's attention, a pivotal step in pharmaceutical advertising. It relies on captivating visuals, compelling headlines, or attention-grabbing health-related statistics. The main goal is to ensure potential customers notice the advertisement and engage with it. In today's media-saturated world, it's essential to act swiftly to catch people's attention, using impactful language or striking imagery that prompts them to pause and explore the content.

During this stage, the primary mission is to capture the attention of potential patients and introduce them to your brand and services. Common content types at this stage include videos, ads, podcasts, and social media posts.

The biggest challenge in this phase is attracting the interest of potential leads. Without them being aware of your existence, meaningful engagement is unlikely. In the digital marketing era, where your target audience is bombarded with numerous marketing messages daily, the question is: How can you make sure your presence stands out amid the competition?

To capture their attention, consider embracing innovative approaches, such as:

1.   Sharing visually striking images with clever, attention-grabbing captions.

2.   Using bold graphics to draw visitors to your website.

3.   Creating engaging, informative videos that introduce prospects to your services.

4.   Incorporating eye-catching visuals into your social media pages.

The goal is to astonish and prompt prospects to pay active attention, but be cautious not to cross the line between cleverness and annoyance.

A message must capture the reader's or viewer's attention almost instantly. Whether through a gripping headline, visually striking elements, or a combination of both, the key is to establish an immediate connection with the audience; without this connection, a message becomes ineffective.

Once the desired audience response is defined, the communicator focuses on crafting an effective message. In traditional marketing terms, the message follows the AIDA model: Attention, Interest, Desire, and Action. However, in pharmaceutical marketing communication, "Desire" is better replaced with "Decision," indicating that the message must not only capture Attention and sustain Interest but also facilitate Decision, ultimately leading to Action—in this case, the issuance of a prescription.

In pharmaceutical marketing, attention is often captured by starting a conversation with a real-life scenario, one that can seamlessly connect with the product's profile. [24] [25] [26]

5.1.2. Interest (I)

After sparking your prospect's interest, the next challenge is retaining it, which can often be more difficult than initially grabbing their attention. You've already ignited curiosity in your target audience, leading them to click a link or watch a video. Now, the question is, how do you keep them engaged?

During this phase of AIDA model marketing, various tools and channels come into play, including website content, TV ads, newsletters, blogs, and email campaigns, all designed to actively involve and captivate potential customers.

The AIDA model is a Proven Technique in Marketing. Sustaining the interest of prospects becomes more manageable when you focus on creating and sharing informative, entertaining videos. Consider maintaining a user-friendly website with concise text paragraphs, highlighted by intriguing headings and dynamic graphics which can be effective in advertising success. [27]

5.1.3. Desire (D)

After establishing initial interest, the focus shifts to nurturing a desire for the pharmaceutical product. This involves persuading potential customers that the medication can effectively address their health needs or improve their quality of life. Pharmaceutical advertisers often emphasize the product's effectiveness, safety, and its potential to deliver positive outcomes for patients. Emotional appeals, such as stories about individuals who have benefited from the medication, can also play a significant role in igniting desire.

Cultivating a desire for your services over those of your competitors is crucial. As you generate interest among your prospects, it becomes essential to explain why your service is superior to your competitors'. This is where you aim to convince your target audience that your service is the solution to their health-related concerns. Naturally, the medication's effectiveness and the level of customer satisfaction after initial use can significantly impact the success of this stage. At this point, the focus should be on showcasing the features and advantages of your service while illustrating how they set you apart from your competitors. Instead of fixating on features, prioritize highlighting the tangible benefits. [28]

5.1.4. Action (A)

After capturing potential customers' attention, keeping them interested, and cultivating desire, the next crucial step is to include a call to action (CTA) that encourages potential patients to schedule an appointment. This can involve placing a direct website link for appointment scheduling, providing an option to sign up for a free consultation, or arranging for your staff to contact prospective clients to understand their needs better. For larger pharmaceutical companies, agencies, distributors, and pharmacies can handle these services.

In essence, the objective here is to persuade potential customers to stop exploring your competitors' websites and make the choice to visit your websites. [29]

[Editor's note: This image had to be removed due to copyright issues.]

Figure 1. Level of the AIDA model

5.2. DAGMAR Model for Pharmaceutical Advertising

The DAGMAR (Defining Advertising Goals for Measured Advertising Results) model serves as a valuable framework in pharmaceutical advertising. By utilizing this model, pharmaceutical advertisers can create campaigns that efficiently communicate the advantages of their medications and prompt the intended actions from their target audience.

Define Objectives: At the core of the DAGMAR model for pharmaceutical advertising lies the imperative task of defining advertising objectives with utmost clarity. Begin by specifying precisely what the campaign aims to achieve. Whether it's raising awareness about a new medication, educating patients on its benefits, or motivating specific behaviors such as consulting a healthcare professional, articulating these objectives serves as the campaign's foundation.

Attainable Goals: Once the objectives are set, the following phase involves defining realistic communication goals. These goals should focus on informing and persuading the target audience. In pharmaceutical advertising, this frequently entails conveying the concrete advantages of the medication, explaining how it works, and addressing patient worries. It's crucial that these goals are both feasible and attainable.

Gauge Success: The DAGMAR model highlights the importance of measuring success using well-defined criteria. To assess the impact of a pharmaceutical advertising campaign, is better to set measurable benchmarks that can be quantified. This may involve tracking selling rates, monitoring patient inquiries, or evaluating changes in patient knowledge and behaviour. These metrics offer a concrete way to evaluate the campaign's effectiveness.

Measure Results: After launching the campaign, it's crucial to diligently measure results against the established criteria. Collect data on key performance indicators (KPIs) to gain insights into the campaign's performance. This step allows for the assessment of the campaign's real-world impact and informs data-driven decisions.

Adapt and Refine: In the dynamic realm of pharmaceutical advertising, adaptability is essential. Based on campaign results and feedback, be prepared to adjust and improve strategies for greater effectiveness. This may involve refining messaging, targeting specific patient demographics more precisely, or optimizing call-to-action elements to encourage desired behaviors.

In conclusion, the DAGMAR model provides a robust framework for pharmaceutical advertisers to plan, execute, and assess their advertising campaigns. By following the principles of clear objective setting, realistic goal establishment, measurable success criteria, and ongoing refinement, pharmaceutical advertisers can effectively convey the value of their medications and prompt desired actions from their target audience in a competitive healthcare landscape. [30] [31]

[Editor's note: This image had to be removed due to copyright issues.]

Figure 2. Level of the Dagmar model

5.3. Rogers' Diffusion

The Rogers' Diffusion of Innovations model is a valuable framework in pharmaceutical advertising. It assists pharmaceutical companies in comprehending and targeting distinct market segments according to their readiness to embrace new medications or treatment methods. Created by Everett M. Rogers in 1962, this model holds particular relevance when introducing new pharmaceutical products to the market.

Here's how the Rogers' Diffusion of Innovations model can be applied in the context of pharmaceutical advertising:

5.3.1. Innovators

Individuals within this category are distinguished by their strong inclination to be trailblazers when it comes to trying out innovations. They have a natural proclivity for exploring uncharted territories and a genuine interest in pioneering ideas. Innovators are inherently inclined to take risks, often leading the way in the development of new concepts. When aiming to reach this demographic, minimal effort is typically required to capture their attention and interest, as their inherent curiosity and inclination for innovation drive their enthusiasm for exploring new pharmaceutical solutions.

In the realm of pharmaceutical products, innovators are at the forefront of early adoption. They typically embody a sense of adventure, readily embracing novel treatments, and often swayed by the latest scientific breakthroughs. When devising pharmaceutical advertising campaigns targeting innovators, the emphasis often revolves around showcasing cutting-edge research, unveiling clinical trial outcomes, and highlighting the medication's novelty.

5.3.2. Early Adopters

In the realm of pharmaceutical adoption, a distinct group of individuals plays a pivotal role as influential opinion leaders. These individuals not only gravitate towards leadership positions but also readily embrace opportunities for change. Remarkably, they possess an inherent awareness of the necessity for change, rendering them highly receptive to the adoption of novel ideas. To effectively resonate with this population, strategies should prioritize the provision of comprehensive how-to manuals and implementation guides. Importantly, this group requires no additional persuasion or information to embrace change.

Closely following the opinion leaders are the early adopters, constituting another substantial segment in the adoption of new pharmaceuticals. These individuals wield influence as opinion leaders within their respective communities and often hold significant sway over the decisions made by others. Pharmaceutical advertisers can effectively capture the attention of early adopters by highlighting the medication's myriad benefits and showcasing how it can profoundly enhance patients' lives.

5.3.3. Early Majority

In the realm of pharmaceutical adoption, a distinctive group embodies the qualities of opinion leaders. These individuals naturally gravitate toward leadership positions and actively seek out opportunities for change. Notably, they possess a keen awareness of the necessity for change, rendering them remarkably receptive to novel concepts. To effectively engage this segment, strategic approaches may include providing comprehensive how-to manuals and informative implementation guides. It's worth emphasizing that this group requires no additional information or persuasion to embrace change.

Conversely, the early majority constitutes a substantial portion of the market and typically adopts new pharmaceuticals once they witness tangible benefits experienced by others. Advertisers can effectively target this segment by showcasing authentic success stories and patient testimonials that underscore the positive outcomes achieved through medication usage.

Therefore, The early adopter is typically held in high regard by their peers and is known for their successful and discreet adoption of new ideas (Rogers, 1971). On the other hand, individuals in the early majority category embrace new ideas just before the typical member of a social system.

5.3.4. Late Majority

Individuals in this category typically approach change with skepticism, choosing to embrace innovation only after it has gained widespread acceptance. To effectively connect with this demographic, strategic efforts should focus on presenting concrete data demonstrating the number of individuals who have not only tried but successfully adopted the innovation.

Conversely, the late majority takes a more cautious and skeptical approach to adopting new medications. Pharmaceutical advertisers should concentrate their efforts on providing comprehensive information regarding safety, efficacy, and the long-term consequences associated with these medications. Addressing the concerns of this group and building trust requires a thorough and transparent approach rooted in data and evidence.

5.3.5. Laggards

Laggards represent the final segment to embrace new pharmaceuticals, often due to their strong resistance to change or deeply ingrained scepticism. Effectively reaching out to laggards may require an alternative approach, focusing on dispelling misconceptions and providing compelling evidence of the medication's tangible benefits. Pharmaceutical advertisers must tailor their messages and marketing strategies to align with the various stages of adoption within the market. This may involve creating educational content, utilizing endorsements from healthcare professionals, conducting informative webinars, or using patient stories to showcase the medication's effectiveness.

Furthermore, pharmaceutical companies should consider the regulatory environment when applying the Rogers' Diffusion of Innovations model. Ensuring that all advertising materials comply with healthcare regulations and guidelines is crucial in this highly regulated industry.

By understanding and adeptly applying the principles of the Rogers' Diffusion of Innovations model, pharmaceutical advertisers can effectively target and engage with different market segments, facilitating the adoption of new medications and ultimately enhancing patient care. [32] [33]

[Editor's note: This image had to be removed due to copyright issues.]

Figure 3: Diffusion of Innovation [34]

It can be said according to the above diagram in figure 3:

Innovators (2.5%) are early adopters who eagerly embrace new ideas and products, often without extensive proof of their effectiveness. They value being at the forefront of innovation and have a strong willingness to explore groundbreaking concepts.

Early Adopters (13.5%): Open to new ideas but need more proof before adopting. Often opinion leaders. Examples: OMD, Mars, Spotify, Microsoft, SC Johnson, Pepsi, Dentsu, ABInBev.

Early Majority (34%): Wait for Early Adopters' approval before trying new innovations. Fear of Missing Out drives their adoption.

Late Majority (34%): Hesitant to change, risk-averse. Only adopt after it's accepted by the Early Majority.

Laggards (16%): Highly resistant to innovation. Prefer old technology and avoid change as long as possible. [35]

6. Advertising Benefits and Harms

Advertising is a ubiquitous part of modern life, influencing our choices, perceptions, and behaviors on a daily basis. It brings both benefits and potential harms to individuals and society as a whole. Let's explore these aspects in more detail:

6.1. Benefits of Pharmaceutical Advertising

Pharmaceutical advertising offers several potential benefits:

6.1.1. Information Dissemination

Information dissemination in pharmaceutical advertising serves several critical functions. Firstly, it acts as a vital tool for conveying essential information about pharmaceutical products, educating healthcare professionals and patients about new treatments, their advantages, and correct usage. Additionally, it can contribute to increased profitability for pharmaceutical companies.

The primary goal of information dissemination is to ensure that the intended audience receives the information effectively. Pharmaceutical advertising not only plays a crucial rôle in successfully introducing new pharmaceutical products but also acts as a vital source of public health information that significantly influences consumer choices and behaviors. However, it's essential to acknowledge that while advertising can boost commercial profitability and raise awareness of medications, it should be closely monitored to prevent self-treatment or improper medical practices. Inappropriate medication promotion, characterized by false or misleading claims, reliance on weak references, and failure to adhere to international standards, can worsen adverse health outcomes. This underscores the importance of government regulations in the pharmaceutical sector to address such issues, as discussed in previous sections. [36]

6.1.2. Patient Empowerment

Patient Patient empowerment is a significant result of well-structured advertising campaigns, providing patients with essential knowledge about their health conditions and available treatment options. Informed patients are better equipped to engage in meaningful conversations with their healthcare providers.

Effective and responsible medication use can directly improve disease outcomes and optimize healthcare resource utilization. Unfortunately, around 50% of patients do not adhere to their prescribed medication regimens, primarily due to a lack of understanding about their medical conditions and the unavailability of reliable medication information.

To enhance public awareness about specific diseases, prescription medications, treatment options, and over-the-counter products, with the ultimate aim of improving patient access to these medications, the concept of "Patient Empowerment" has emerged as an innovative approach. This approach seeks to strengthen public knowledge about diseases, medications, and their appropriate usage, while also advancing medical awareness and encouraging patient adherence to prescribed treatments. [37]

6.1.3. Disease Awareness

Pharmaceutical advertising plays a crucial role in increasing awareness of specific medical conditions, reducing associated stigmas, and encouraging individuals to seek diagnosis and treatment. While previous research has primarily examined how disease awareness advertising affects the relationship between Pharmaceutical manufacturers and consumers, it is equally important to consider the perspectives of healthcare professionals, particularly physicians, who have a significant role in the healthcare sector.

Study results indicate that the majority of physicians hold positive views regarding disease awareness advertising. These findings underscore that disease awareness advertising can improve public awareness of diseases and medications, especially over-the-counter (OTC) medications, which can promote responsible medication use. However, there are differing opinions about its impact on patients. Some physicians express concerns that disease awareness advertising may lead to patient confusion and unwarranted fear. Additionally, a notable suggestion is made that disease awareness advertising should be conducted in collaboration with non-profit organizations to mitigate the perception of commercial interests associated with pharmaceutical companies that sponsor these awareness campaigns. [38]

6.1.4. Market Competition

Research Research has shown that effective promotion of over-the-counter (OTC) products by pharmaceutical companies depends on the products adhering to quality, safety, and performance standards outlined in regulatory requirements. Such adherence not only creates a lasting brand image in consumers' minds but also fosters competitiveness in the market. The primary goal of OTC advertising is to inform the public about their health conditions and the availability of personalized medical solutions, thereby enhancing market competition.

Considering that consumer product advertising is constrained by the amount of information that can be conveyed, its role primarily revolves around capturing attention and fostering appreciation in a highly competitive environment. Additional communication channels, such as product labels and brochures, play a crucial role in providing comprehensive information and further strengthening a product's competitive edge. Advertising for registered medications offers numerous advantages for public health, the overall market, and individual patients, contributing to increased competition among pharmaceutical companies.

Pharmaceutical companies can effectively promote their products in the market when their offerings align with safety, efficacy, and brand recognition in consumers' minds. To achieve and maintain a competitive edge, pharmaceutical companies must employ compelling and engaging marketing strategies to distinguish their products from competitors in the market. Establishing strong relationships with pharmacists and healthcare professionals is essential not only for long-term success but also for cultivating a positive perception of their products among consumers, further fueling competition within the industry. Sustainability in the market can be achieved through well-planned promotional and marketing strategies that adapt to the evolving landscape of information proliferation, technological advancements, and heightened competition, ensuring a strong competitive presence for pharmaceutical companies. [39]

6.1.5. Economic Impact

Pharmaceutical advertising wields a substantial and multifaceted economic influence. It has the potential to bolster sales, broaden markets, generate employment opportunities, stimulate research and development, and encourage competition within the industry. Nevertheless, its impact on healthcare costs and resource allocation may also rise, contingent on how it shapes patients' choices and healthcare providers' decisions. Successful advertising initiatives can cultivate brand loyalty, thereby securing a consistent revenue flow for pharmaceutical enterprises. The comprehensive economic consequences are contingent upon several factors, encompassing the efficacy of advertising campaigns and the regulatory framework in place. [40]

6.2 Harms of Pharmaceutical Advertising

Pharmaceutical advertising also carries potential risks and harms:

6.2.1. Misleading Information

Some Certain advertisements have the tendency to overstate the advantages of a medication while minimizing its associated risks, consequently promoting misinformation and potentially inappropriate utilization.

Misleading pharmaceutical advertising can have adverse consequences on both consumers and the healthcare system. Past research has shown that medication advertisements directed at physicians can be misleading. Nevertheless, there exists a scarcity of research comparing consumer-targeted pharmaceutical advertising to available evidence, thereby hindering the assessment of the presence of misleading or false information in these advertisements. [41]

6.2.2. Overmedicalization

Aggressive advertising can contribute to overmedicalization, where individuals seek unnecessary treatments or medications.

6.2.3. Increased Healthcare Costs

The marketing expenses associated with pharmaceutical advertising can contribute to higher medication prices and overall healthcare costs.

6.2.4. Ethical Concerns

Ethical concerns arise when advertisements prioritize profits over patient well-being, potentially compromising the doctor-patient relationship. [42]

7. The Landscape of Over-the-Counter (OTC) medications in Hungary

A study conducted in Hungary aimed to assess pharmacists' perspectives on over-the-counter (OTC) medication advertisements and their informative value. The findings indicated that over 70% of pharmacists observed that patients possess only a basic understanding of OTC medications. Moreover, approximately 50-70% of the population requests OTC medications by specific names.

Notably, residents of Budapest exhibit greater familiarity with OTC medicines compared to those in smaller settlements, possibly due to enhanced access to information. Younger patients, influenced by parental guidance, advertising, and the internet, tend to be more receptive to medication information, while individuals aged 65 and above may encounter challenges in accessing such information.

Gender differences are also observed, with women displaying a higher willingness to embrace new medications and heed pharmacy recommendations. Provincial pharmacies often receive more consultation requests and can allocate additional time to each patient. Reward systems that value pharmaceutical care align with patients' willingness to pay for such services. Of course, the advantages and rewards of pharmaceutical companies over pharmacies can be effective in introducing OTC medications to patients.

In general, the study reveals that people often lack an in-depth understanding of OTC medications and frequently base their decisions on advertisements, which may not consistently yield the desired results. Patients increasingly expect professional guidance and care from pharmacists, emphasizing the importance of comprehensive medication explanations, accurate dosage instructions, and nurturing positive patient-pharmacist relationships. Furthermore, it is crucial to educate the public about the significance of seeking professional advice when purchasing OTC medications, rather than relying solely on advertisements. The development of effective self-medication algorithms and improved technology for linking pharmacy and physician databases are essential in enhancing patient care. Pharmacists must excel in communication, be well-versed in advertising techniques, and possess a deep understanding of the psychology of persuasion. [43] [44]

8. Discussion

Advertising within the pharmaceutical industry is expansive in scope. Building upon the insights presented in earlier sections, we can succinctly summarize the discussion on pharmaceutical advertising in this section.

The exploration of pharmaceutical advertising benefits and harms in this study reveals a multifaceted landscape where advertising's impact transcends mere promotion. While it has the potential to provide valuable information, empower patients, and drive innovation, it also carries the risk of misinformation, overmedicalization, and increased healthcare costs. Balancing these advantages and disadvantages remains a central challenge for both the pharmaceutical industry and regulatory authorities.

The historical evolution of pharmaceutical advertising, as outlined in Section 2, sheds light on the intricate relationship between advances in communication, societal shifts, and the ethical responsibilities of pharmaceutical companies. From ancient methods of sharing medical wisdom to the modern era of highly regulated advertising, this evolution underscores the ongoing tension between disseminating valuable medical information and the potential for misinformation or undue influence.

One key takeaway from this historical perspective is the importance of striking a balance between accessibility and accuracy. While early forms of medical advertising lacked scientific rigor, they laid the groundwork for more responsible and regulated practices in the modern era. The emergence of regulatory bodies, such as the FDA in the United States and similar agencies in other countries, underscores the need for oversight to ensure that pharmaceutical advertising aligns with medical ethics and delivers accurate information.

The discussion of pharmaceutical advertising regulations, both at the European Union level and within Hungary, highlights the complexity of navigating advertising guidelines in a global industry. While EU directives provide a broad framework, individual member states, like Hungary, have the flexibility to adapt regulations to their specific contexts. This variability necessitates a nuanced understanding of regional requirements when crafting pharmaceutical advertising campaigns. The mentioned laws in Hungary aim to protect consumer interests, promote fair market practices, and address unfair trade activities. They emphasize the importance of self-regulation and codes of conduct within the relevant industries. These laws cover various aspects of advertising and commercial practices, including those related to pharmaceuticals. They govern practices throughout the entire commercial process, from advertising to post-transaction activities. These regulations apply to commercial practices within Hungary and those affecting consumers in the country, contributing significantly to consumer protection and the maintenance of fair and ethical business practices.

The application of advertising models like AIDA and DAGMAR in pharmaceutical advertising underscores the significance of effective communication in the industry. These models help advertisers navigate the intricate path of conveying information about pharmaceutical products to various audiences. However, they also emphasize the responsibility to provide accurate, balanced, and ethical messaging, especially when dealing with matters of health and well-being.

The Rogers' Diffusion of Innovations model offers valuable insights into how pharmaceutical advertisers can approach different segments of the market based on their readiness to adopt new medications. Recognizing that not all consumers are early adopters underscores the need for tailored messaging and educational content to address varying levels of skepticism and readiness for change.

In conclusion, this study underscores the complexities and nuances of pharmaceutical advertising, both historically and in the contemporary landscape. Striking a balance between the benefits and potential harms of pharmaceutical advertising requires vigilance, ethical responsibility, and adherence to regulatory guidelines. The responsible communication of medical information is paramount in an industry where health and well-being are at stake.

9. Conclusion

Pharmaceutical advertising is a dynamic and complex field that has evolved significantly throughout history. From ancient oral traditions to modern, highly regulated campaigns, the industry has witnessed profound changes in how medical information is communicated to the public. This evolution reflects the ongoing quest for balance between accessibility, accuracy, and ethics in healthcare communication.

Regulatory frameworks, both at the EU and national levels, play a crucial role in shaping the responsible conduct of pharmaceutical advertising. These regulations serve as safeguards to ensure that promotional materials meet rigorous standards of accuracy and ethics. Advertisers must navigate this intricate web of guidelines to promote their products effectively while adhering to ethical principles. Pharmaceutical advertising regulations in the EU and Hungary are complex due to variations in regional requirements. Hungary's laws aim to protect consumers, promote fairness, and combat unfair trade practices, aligning with broader EU directives. In summary, understanding these regulations is vital for crafting effective and compliant pharmaceutical advertising campaigns.

Advertising models, such as AIDA, DAGMAR, and the Rogers' Diffusion of Innovations model, offer pharmaceutical companies valuable tools to engage with diverse audiences. These models emphasize the importance of clear communication, measurable objectives, and tailored messaging to meet the varying needs and attitudes of consumers.

In this era of rapid technological advancement and global information dissemination, pharmaceutical advertising continues to hold immense potential to inform, educate, and empower healthcare consumers. However, with this potential comes the ethical responsibility to prioritize patient well-being and provide transparent and accurate information.

As pharmaceutical advertising continues to evolve, it is essential for both industry professionals and regulatory bodies to collaborate in fostering an environment where responsible communication of medical information, informed decision-making, and patient empowerment take centre stage. By doing so, we can ensure that pharmaceutical advertising remains a force for good in the healthcare landscape, ultimately benefiting the well-being of individuals and society. Following the completion of a questionnaire among pharmacists and patients, it is evident that a unanimous positive consensus exists regarding the impact of advertising on non-prescription medications. The questionnaire itself will be included in the subsequent section.

10.   Questionnaire

A questionnaire was administered to ten pharmacists and patients to gather their opinions on pharmaceutical advertising. The questionnaire and the results are as follows:

Question 1: Should advertising of medicines be allowed?

Yes: (100%)

No: (0%)

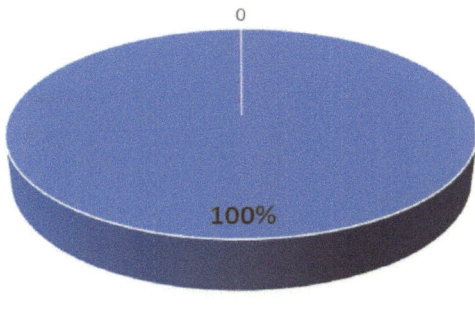

Question 1

Question 2: Which factors influence a consumer's decision to buy a medicine?

Brand name (30%)

Price: (30%)

Advertised benefits: (20%)

Doctor's recommendation (20%)

Side effects: 0 respondents (0%)

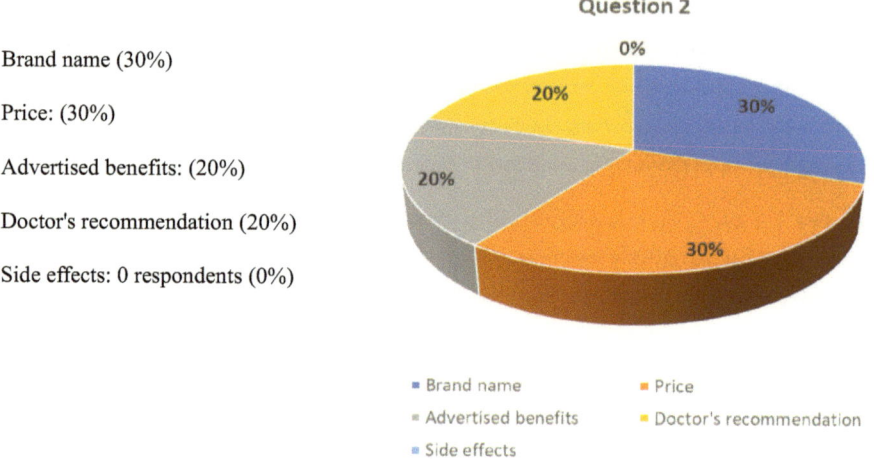

Question 3: Which type of advertising is most effective in promoting medicines?

Television commercials: (50%)

Social media: (20%)

Billboards: (10%)

In-store displays: (10%)

Print ads: (10%)

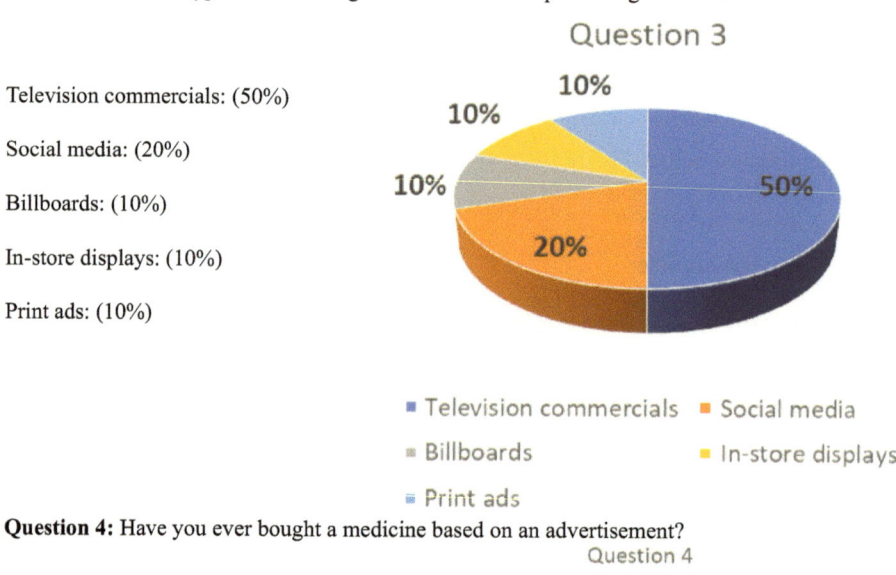

Question 4: Have you ever bought a medicine based on an advertisement?

Yes: (100%)

No: (0%)

Question 5: How do you feel about the use of fear tactics in medicine advertisements? (Rate on a scale of 0 to 10, with 0 being strongly dislike and 10 being strongly like)

Average rating: 7.2

Responses varied from 2 to 10, indicating mixed feelings.

Question 6: Do you think that the side effects of a medicine should be included in its advertisement?

Yes: (100%)

No: (0%)

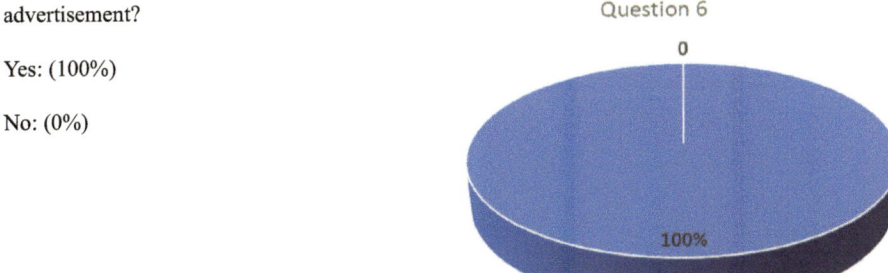

Question 7: If yes, how much emphasis should be given to the side effects?

A lot: (50%)

Some: (50%)

A little: (0%)

None: (0%)

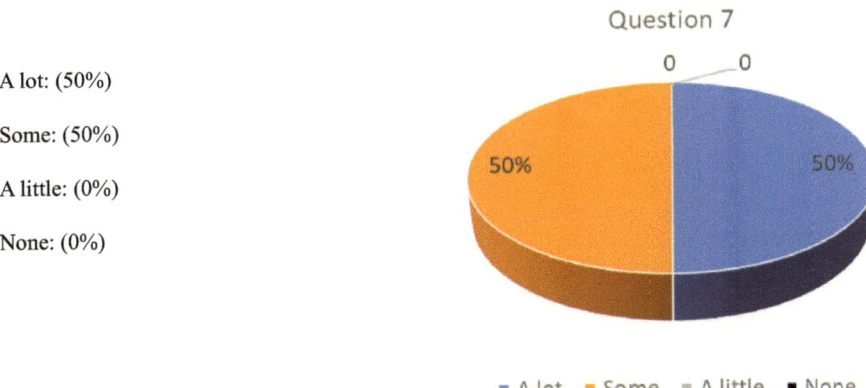

Question 8: Which appeals do you think are most effective in medicine advertisements?

Emotional appeal: (28.6%)

Rational appeal: (57.1%)

Celebrity endorsement: (42.9%)

Humor: (57.1%)

Scarcity: (42.9%)

These findings give us a better understanding of what the participants think about pharmaceutical ads. It includes their likes and feelings about different parts of these ads.

Acknowledgment

I extend my heartfelt appreciation to the teachers and staff at the University of Szeged, Pharmacy Department and especially Dr. Háznagyné Dr. Radnai Erzsébet. Your guidance and expertise have played a pivotal role in shaping my research and academic growth. I am truly grateful for your unwavering support throughout the course of my education.

References

[1] [Online]. Available: https://www.pharmacytimes.com/view/the-evolving-world-of-pharma-marketing.

[2] [Online]. Available: https://www.britannica.com/science/history-of-medicine.

[3] [Online]. Available: https://blogs.library.duke.edu/digital-collections/mma/about/.

[4] [Online]. Available: https://industrialrevolutionspod.com/episodes/2019/12/17/chapter-38-the-advent-of-modern-advertising.

[5] Mackey, T. K., Cuomo, R. E., & Liang, B. A. (2015). The rise of digital direct-to-consumer advertising?: Comparison of direct-to-consumer advertising expenditure trends from publicly available data sources and global policy implications. In BMC Health Services Research (Vol. 15, Issue 1). Springer Science and Business Media LLC. https://doi.org/10.1186/s12913-015-0885-1

[6] "DONOHUE, J. (2006). A History of Medication Advertising: The Evolving Roles of Consumers and Consumer Protection. In The Milbank Quarterly (Vol. 84, Issue 4, pp. 659–699). Wiley. https://doi.org/10.1111/j.1468-0009.2006.00464.x

[7] [Online]. Available: https://blue-reg.com/news/pharmaceutical-advertising-regulations-in-europe-responsible-persons/.

[8] [Online]. Available: https://www.euvolution.com/futurist-transhuman-news-blog/food-supplements/an-overview-of-eu-rules-on-consumer-advertising-of-over-the-counter-products-in-the-life-sciences-sector-media-telecoms-it-entertainment.php.

[9] [Online]. Available: https://www.europarl.europa.eu/meetdocs/2004_2009/documents/pr/729/729812/729812en.pdf.

[10] [Online]. Available: https://health.ec.europa.eu/system/files/2016-11/beuc_e.

[11] [Online]. Available: https://www.nnk.gov.hu/.

[12] [Online]. Available: https://ogyei.gov.hu/figyelemfelhivas_tovabbi_hatosagi_ugyintezesre.

[13] [Online]. Available: https://www.nnk.gov.hu/index.php/nnk-hirek/2096-osszevonjak-nnk-ogyei.

[14] [Online]. Available: https://www.nnk.gov.hu/.

[15] [Online]. Available: https://ogyei.gov.hu/figyelemfelhivas_tovabbi_hatosagi_ugyintezesre.

[16] [Online]. Available: https://medicalonline.hu/eu_gazdasag/cikk/megkezdi_a_munkat_a_nemzeti_nepegeszsegugyi_kozpont.

[17] [Online]. Available: https://nepszava.hu/3017097_megvan-az-uj-tisztifoorvos.

[18] [Online]. Available: https://net.jogtar.hu/jogszabaly?docid=a0600098.tv&dbnum=62&getdoc=1.

[19] [Online]. Available: https://net.jogtar.hu/getpdf?docid=a0600098.tv&targetdate=&printTitle=Act+XCVIII+of+2006&dbnum=62&getdoc=1.

[20] [Online]. Available: https://net.jogtar.hu/jogszabaly?docid=a0900003.eum.

[21] [Online]. Available: https://net.jogtar.hu/jogszabaly?docid=a0800048.tv.

[22] [Online]. Available: https://www.gvh.hu/data/cms998396/jogihatter_jogszab_gyujt_Grtv_2008_m%C3%B3d_09_4_jav.pdf.

[23] [Online]. Available: https://net.jogtar.hu/jogszabaly?docid=a0800047.tv.

https://cms.law/en/int/expert-guides/cms-expert-guide-to-advertising-of-medicines-and-medical-devices/hungary

[24] [Online]. Available: https://www.practicebuilders.com/blog/aida-marketing-a-proven-technique-to-convert-prospects-into-patients/.

[25] [Online]. Available: https://healthcaresuccess.com/blog/advertising/remember-aida-engaging-your-medical-marketing-audience-simplified.html.

[26] [Online]. Available: https://www.thepharmajournal.com/vol3Issue5/Issue_july_2014/18.1.pdf.

[27] [Online]. Available: https://www.practicebuilders.com/blog/aida-marketing-a-proven-technique-to-convert-prospects-into-patients/.

[28] [Online]. Available: https://www.practicebuilders.com/blog/aida-marketing-a-proven-technique-to-convert-prospects-into-patients/.

[29] [Online]. Available: https://www.practicebuilders.com/blog/aida-marketing-a-proven-technique-to-convert-prospects-into-patients/.

[30] [Online]. Available: https://www.investopedia.com/terms/d/dagmar.asp.

[31] [Online]. Available: https://www.marketing91.com/dagmar/.

[32] [Online]. Available: https://sphweb.bumc.bu.edu/otlt/mph-modules/sb/behavioralchangetheories/behavioralchangetheories4.html.

[33] Dearing, J. W., & Cox, J. G. (2018). Diffusion Of Innovations Theory, Principles, And Practice. In Health Affairs (Vol. 37, Issue 2, pp. 183–190). Health Affairs (Project Hope). https://doi.org/10.1377/hlthaff.2017.1104

[34] [Online]. Available: https://the-media-leader.com/attention-revolution-crossing-the-audience-measurement-chasm/.

[35] [Online]. Available: https://the-media-leader.com/attention-revolution-crossing-the-audience-measurement-chasm/.

[36] Yousefi, N., Sharif, Z., Chahian, F., Mombeini, T., & Peiravian, F. (2022). An investigation into the pharmaceutical advertising in Iranian medical journals. In Journal of Pharmaceutical Policy and Practice (Vol. 15, Issue 1). Springer Science and Business Media LLC. https://doi.org/10.1186/s40545-022-00415-1

[37] Schwartzberg, E., Barnett-Itzhaki, Z., Grotto, I., & Marom, E. (2017). Strategies for patient empowerment through the promotion of medicines in Israel: regulatory framework for the pharmaceutical industry. In Israel Journal of Health Policy Research (Vol. 6, Issue 1). Springer Science and Business Media LLC. https://doi.org/10.1186/s13584-017-0175-y

[38] Banerjee, S., & Dash, S. K. (2013). Effectiveness of disease awareness advertising in emerging economy: Views of health care professionals of India. In Journal of Medical Marketing: Device, Diagnostic and Pharmaceutical Marketing (Vol. 13, Issue 4, pp. 231–241). SAGE Publications. https://doi.org/10.1177/1745790413516479

[39] [Online]. Available: https://www.ijcrt.org/papers/IJCRT2104318.pdf.

[40] Z. J. L. (. by Stuart O. Schweitzer (Author), Pharmaceutical Economics and Policy: Perspectives, Promises, and Problems 3rd Edition.

[41] Faerber, A. E., & Kreling, D. H. (2013). Content Analysis of False and Misleading Claims in Television Advertising for Prescription and Nonprescription Drugs. In Journal of General Internal Medicine (Vol. 29, Issue 1, pp. 110–118). Springer Science and Business Media LLC. https://doi.org/10.1007/s11606-013-2604-0

[42] Hanslik, T., & Flahault, A. (2016). Overmedicalization: when too much medicine harms your health. In The Journal of Internal Medicine (Vol. 37, Issue 3, pp. 201–205). Elsevier BV. DOI: 10.1016/j.revmed.2015.10.009

[Online]. Available: https://www.nbcnews.com/health/health-news/health-care-industry-spends-30-billion-year-marketing-n956251

[43] Major, C., & Vincze, Z. (2010). Consumer habits and interests regarding non-prescription medications in Hungary. In Family Practice (Vol. 27, Issue 3, pp. 333–338). Oxford University Press (OUP). https://doi.org/10.1093/fampra/cmp105

[44] [Online]. Available: https://www.ptfarm.pl/pub/File/Acta_Poloniae/2010/5/547.pdf.

[45] "https://www.pharmacytimes.com/view/the-evolving-world-of-pharma-marketing," [Online].

[46] [Online]. Available: https://health.ec.europa.eu/system/files/2016-11/beuc_e.

[47] [Online]. Available: https://www.practicebuilders.com/blog/aida-marketing-a-proven-technique-to-convert-prospects-into-patients/.

YOUR KNOWLEDGE HAS VALUE

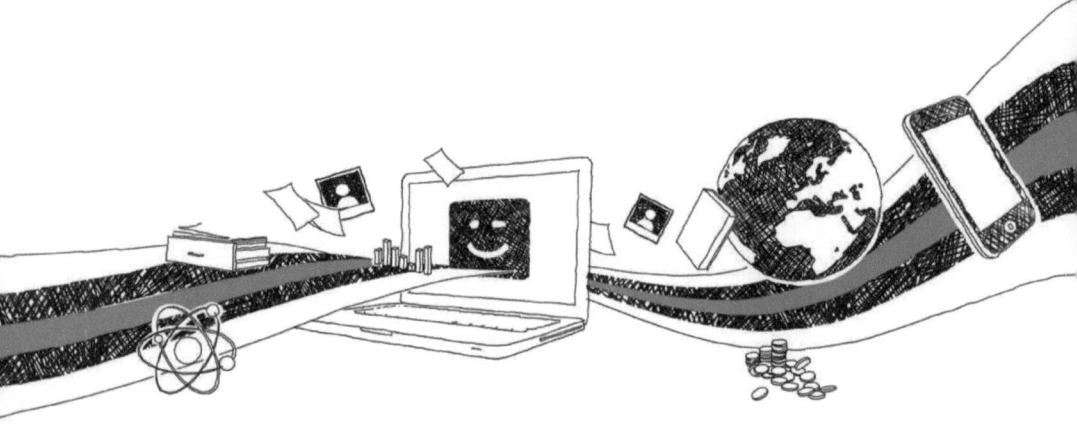

- We will publish your bachelor's and
  master's thesis, essays and papers

- Your own eBook and book -
  sold worldwide in all relevant shops

- Earn money with each sale

Upload your text at www.GRIN.com
and publish for free

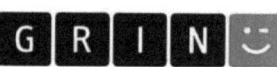